EVERYTHING ABOUT

ALKALINE DIET

Secret To Vibrant Living On Whole Food Diet, Complete Alkaline Recipe Cookbook For Weight Loss And Health Improvement

DR. ALVIN BRANTLEY

Disclaimer

The information provided in this book is intended for general informational purposes only. It is not a substitute for professional medical advice, diagnosis, or treatment.

You should not use the information in this book for diagnosing or treating a health problem or disease by self decision. Always seek the advice of your physician or other qualified health provider with any questions you may have regarding a medical condition.

The author and publisher of this book make no representations or warranties with respect to the accuracy, applicability, fitness, or completeness of the contents of this book. The information contained in this book is based on the author's research and experience, and it is shared with the understanding that the author is not engaged in rendering medical, health, or any other kind of professional advice for you by this book.

The author does not endorse or promote any specific products, brands, or companies related to the contents provided in this book.

Any mention of products or services in this book is for informational purposes only and does not constitute an endorsement.

The author has not entered into any affiliate marketing agreements and has not signed any endorsement deals with individuals, organizations, or companies.

Readers are encouraged to consult with their healthcare providers before making any dietary or lifestyle chaSnges based on the information provided in this book. The author and publisher disclaim any liability for the decisions made by readers based on the information in this book.

Contents

The Introduction Of An Alkaline Diet

The Alkaline Diet has become well-known as a dietary strategy for preserving the pH equilibrium of the body.

This diet's proponents contend that eating foods that increase alkalinity will help the body reach a more ideal pH level, which will enhance health and well-being.

Examining the physics underlying pH balance as well as the fundamentals of the alkaline diet are necessary to comprehend its foundation.

CHAPTER ONE

What Diet Is Alkaline?

The foundation of the alkaline diet, sometimes referred to as the acid-alkaline diet or the alkaline ash diet, is the idea of bringing the body's pH levels into balance. To offset the acidity that can arise from the standard Western diet, this diet places a strong emphasis on consuming foods that are alkaline-forming. Foods that are alkaline-forming are thought to balance out too much acid in the body and make it more alkaline overall.

The pH Scale Explained

It's important to understand the pH scale to understand the Alkaline Diet. The pH scale, which goes from 0 to 14 and considers 7 to be neutral, is used to quantify acidity or alkalinity.

An alkaline pH is greater than 7, and an acidic pH is less than 7. The pH range that the human body aims to maintain is roughly 7.35 to 7.45, which is slightly alkaline. The goal of the alkaline diet is to assist the body in preserving this delicate pH equilibrium.

Alkaline Vs. Acidic Foods

An essential component of the Alkaline Diet is knowing which foods are acidic and alkaline. Acidic foods often increase the body's acidity, which may cause health problems.

However, it's crucial to remember that meals are classified as acidic or alkaline based on the residue they leave in the body after digestion. On the other hand, alkaline-forming foods are thought to counteract acidity and encourage a more alkaline pH.

Foods With High Acidity To Avoid

Limiting the consumption of items rich in acidity is emphasized in the Alkaline Diet. These consist of refined carbohydrates, processed foods, and some animal products. It is believed that consuming fewer of these foods will help keep the body from being overly acidic, improving general health.

Typical foods that are rich in acidity include dairy, meat, coffee, and some grains.

Foods That Form Alkaloids To Incorporate

In contrast, the Alkaline Diet promotes the consumption of foods that generate an alkaline environment in the body.

Typically, these foods include grains, nuts, seeds, fruits, and vegetables.

The Alkaline Diet's proponents contend that by promoting the body's natural pH equilibrium, a diet high in certain foods might improve health.

The core principle of the alkaline diet is to use food to keep the body's pH level in check.

Although there is little scientific proof to back up the Alkaline Diet's claims, some people find it to be good for their general health.

Before making any major dietary changes, it is imperative to speak with a healthcare provider, just like with any diet.

The Science Of Ph Equilibrium

The idea behind pH balancing is to keep the body's acid-base balance intact. pH is a measurement of how acidic or alkaline a substance is.

The pH scale has a range of 0 to 14, with 7 being neutral and 14 being extremely alkaline. The ideal pH for the body is 7.4, which is a little bit on the alkaline side to support certain physiological activities.

CHAPTER TWO

The Impact Of Ph On The Body

The pH balance of the body is essential for general health and well-being. Various physiological systems and processes function best within particular pH ranges.

Enzymes, for example, are sensitive to pH variations and are necessary for a variety of biological activities.

A pH variation from ideal levels might impact the action of enzymes, causing disturbances in metabolic processes and jeopardizing cellular operations.

Acidic environments can cause inflammation, harm to cells, and heightened susceptibility to illnesses. On the other hand, preserving a slightly alkaline pH is thought to provide an atmosphere that is favorable to optimum health, encouraging improved cellular function and general well-being.

Alkalinity And The Prevention Of Diseases

The foundation of the alkaline diet is the idea that eating foods that generate an alkaline environment aids in preserving the pH balance of the body, which helps ward against illness.

Alkaline diet proponents contend that an excessively acidic internal environment may play a role in the emergence of chronic illnesses like diabetes, cardiovascular disease, and osteoporosis.

Fruits, vegetables, and some grains are considered alkaline-rich foods because they counteract acidity and promote a more alkaline pH.

People who include these items in their diet are said to be less likely to suffer from various health problems and to feel better overall.

Methods For Testing Ph

There are several testing techniques available to monitor and control pH levels.

By offering information on the body's acid-alkaline balance, these techniques help people make well-informed food decisions.

Ph Testing Of Urine

One popular technique for determining the body's acidity or alkalinity is urine pH testing. The pH level of urine is measured using pH strips in this non-invasive method.

A pH of 6.5 to 7.5 is generally regarded as normal. Variations from this range could be a sign of abnormalities in the acid-base balance of the body, leading people to modify their diet to create a more alkaline environment.

Saliva Ph Measurement

Another technique used to assess the pH balance of the body is saliva pH testing. This method uses pH strips to measure acidity or alkalinity, much like urine pH testing. Saliva pH monitoring, according to proponents of the alkaline diet, can reveal important details about the general health of the body.

Opponents counter that saliva pH can be influenced by things like recent food consumption and dental cleanliness, which could result in less reliable results than with other testing techniques.

To maintain optimal health, it is imperative to comprehend the science underlying pH balance.

The goal of the alkaline diet is to encourage the body to have a slightly alkaline environment by emphasizing the consumption of foods that generate an alkaline state.

Tests for pH, such as those that measure the pH of saliva and urine, give people the ability to keep an eye on their acid-base balance and make decisions that will benefit their general health.

CHAPTER THREE

Creating An Alkaline Dietary Program

Keeping the body's pH level in balance is crucial for general health, and eating an alkaline diet is one way to accomplish this.

To offset the acidity that can arise from contemporary dietary choices, an alkaline diet mainly concentrates on eating foods that support an alkaline environment in the body.

This article will walk you through creating an alkaline diet plan, including meal planning tips, alkaline breakfast ideas, alkaline lunch recipes, alkaline dinner selections, and an exploration of alkaline snack options.

Organizing Your Dinners

Meal planning is essential when starting an alkaline diet. The secret is to minimize your intake of acidic foods like processed meals, dairy products, and some grains and to include a variety of alkaline-forming foods like fruits, vegetables, nuts, and seeds.

Maintaining an ideal pH level in the body through balancing acidic and alkaline foods promotes general health.

Ideas For Alkaline Breakfasts

Eating an alkaline meal in the morning creates a favorable environment for preserving pH equilibrium during the day. Think about including fruits high in alkaloids, such as citrus, melons, and berries, in your daily routine.

You may make your breakfast even more alkaline by serving these fruits with grains that are high in minerals, like amaranth or quinoa.

Furthermore, leafy green smoothies made with spinach or kale might be a great option for an alkalizing and nutrient-rich start to the day.

Alkaline Meal Ideas

You can further assist your alkaline aims at lunch. Choose salads that are abundant in alkaline vegetables, like bell peppers, cucumbers, and broccoli. Incorporate protein-rich foods that promote an alkaline environment, such as legumes or tofu. You can experiment with flavor-enhancing alkaline dressings that contain lemon, olive oil, and herbs without sacrificing the pH equilibrium.

Alkaline Supper Ideas

Incorporate a variety of vegetables, especially leafy greens and cruciferous vegetables, for a well-rounded alkaline supper.

Alkaline grains like brown rice or quinoa can be used with lean protein sources like fish or plant-based substitutes. It's best to avoid eating too many acidic sauces and condiments because they can make the body more acidic.

Maintaining an alkaline diet involves snacking. To sate desires between meals, go for alkaline snacks like raw almonds, seeds, or fresh fruit.

Make sure that the snacks you choose help to the overall alkaline balance by avoiding processed foods and choosing homemade alternatives.

Water To Maintain Ph Balance

One essential component of pH balance is hydration. Although water has no inherent acidity, different kinds of water can affect how acidic the body is. Selecting alkaline water, which generally has a higher pH, can help keep the pH level in the body at its ideal level.

Maintaining adequate hydration is crucial for general health and supports the benefits of an alkaline diet.

Advantages Of Alkaline Water

Because of its possible advantages in fostering pH equilibrium, alkaline water has grown in popularity.

Alkaline water's proponents contend that it has antioxidant qualities and can balance the body's acidity.

While further research is needed to confirm these claims, adding alkaline water to your daily hydration regimen can help you achieve pH equilibrium overall.

Strategic meal planning, with a focus on alkaline-forming foods, is essential to creating and adhering to an alkaline diet plan.

Selecting alkaline-rich foods throughout the day, from breakfast to dinner and snacks in between, helps to create a more alkaline environment in the body, which enhances general health and well-being.

In the search for pH balance, being aware of hydration—especially with alkaline water—can support these nutritional efforts.

CHAPTER FOUR

Alkaline Daily Activities

Sustaining an alkaline lifestyle is essential to attaining the ideal pH equilibrium in the body.

To balance out the acidic content of many modern diets, the alkaline diet emphasizes consuming foods that support an alkaline environment.

In this nutritional strategy, fruits and vegetables—especially those with a high alkaline content—are essential.

Through the use of foods high in alkali, people want to establish an environment within themselves that promotes overall health.

Including Exercise To Maintain Ph Balance

Getting regular exercise is essential for maintaining the body's pH equilibrium. Exercise is beneficial to overall health and helps keep the body in an alkaline state.

Exercises that improve circulation, oxygenation, and the body's ability to eliminate acidic waste products include yoga, strength training, and cardiovascular exercises.

An alkaline diet and a well-rounded fitness program work together to create an environment that is favorable to pH homeostasis.

One frequent element that has a big effect on the body's pH levels is stress. Prolonged stress causes the hormone cortisol, which is linked to acidity, to be released.

The acidifying effects of stress can be lessened by incorporating stress management approaches such as deep breathing exercises, mindfulness training, and meditation.

Through stress management and relaxation techniques, people can help maintain an alkaline pH, which promotes general health and vitality.

The body needs good sleep to carry out its normal functions, which include regulating pH.

The body regenerates and repairs itself as we sleep, which affects the overall acid-alkaline balance.

The body's capacity to sustain an alkaline state can be improved by establishing regular sleep schedules and furnishing a comfortable sleeping space

Sufficient and peaceful sleep enhances other alkaline living practices, creating a comprehensive strategy for maintaining pH equilibrium and general health.

Detoxification Methodologies

An essential part of living an alkaline lifestyle is detoxification, which helps the body get rid of waste items that have become acidic over time.

A variety of detoxification techniques, including sauna sessions, herbal cleanses, and intermittent fasting, help to eliminate toxins and support pH balance.

These methods support the liver and kidneys, two organs involved in detoxification, by lowering the body's acidic burden.

By including detoxification in the alkaline lifestyle, the body becomes more resistant to acidity.

Smoothies with an alkaline detox are a tasty and practical approach to increase alkalinity and aid the body's natural detoxification processes.

Alkaline-rich fruits and vegetables, like citrus fruits, berries, and leafy greens, are frequently used in these smoothies.

Supplementing with chia, flax, or spirulina seeds might intensify their alkalizing effects.

Smoothies with an alkaline detox contribute vital nutrients and help maintain pH balance, making them a revitalizing and nourishing complement to an alkaline diet.

Including these smoothies regularly might be a tasty and practical way to keep your lifestyle alkaline.

CHAPTER FIVE

Common Misconceptions And Myths

The principle behind the alkaline diet is that particular meals can change the pH levels of the body by making it more acidic or alkaline.

However, there are a lot of false beliefs and fallacies about this eating strategy.

The idea that eating alkaline foods may rapidly and substantially alter the body's pH is one of the most widespread misconceptions.

In actuality, the body has an extremely complex buffering system that controls pH levels to preserve a stable internal environment.

The idea that all acidic meals are unhealthy is another common misperception.

Some acidic foods might indeed make the body more acidic, but not all acidic foods have the same impact.

Citrus fruits, for example, once they are digested, can have an alkalizing impact despite their acidity. Differentiating between a food's pH before digestion and its effect on the pH of the body following digestion is crucial.

Dispelling Myths About Alkaline Diets

Clarity on the alkaline diet is achieved by addressing and debunking prevalent myths. One common misconception is that the secret to good health is to follow an exclusively alkaline diet. In actuality, it is usually advised to have a diversified and balanced diet that consists of a combination of foods that generate acid and alkaline. Nutritional imbalances and deficits can result from eating only alkaline meals and avoiding all acidic ones.

Furthermore, the alkaline diet is frequently linked to weight loss; some people even swear that it may magically eliminate extra pounds. While eating a diet high in fruits and vegetables can help control weight, it is oversimplified to attribute weight loss to food's alkaline properties alone. Many elements go into keeping a healthy weight.

Drinking alkaline water is one part of the alkaline diet that has received attention. Alkaline water proponents contend that it can balance the body's acidity and offer several health advantages.

Nevertheless, a rigorous analysis of this assertion demonstrates a lack of agreement among scientists.

The pH can be stabilized by the body's natural buffering mechanisms, and research is still being done to determine the effects of alkaline water on general health.

Certain critics contend that the promotion of alkaline water as a panacea for many health concerns could be deceptive. The human body is flexible and can adjust to many different food regimens. While being hydrated is important for good health, alkaline water alone may not address all of the issues associated with health, including lifestyle, exercise, and general food.

Busting Myths About Ph

Understanding the body's complex pH-regulating systems is crucial to dispelling myths about pH and its effects on health. The blood's pH is kept by the body slightly alkaline, usually between 7.35 and 7.45. Enzymes and other biological activities depend on this small pH range to function properly.

Diet has little effect on blood pH, but it can affect urine pH.

Dispelling myths about pH levels requires highlighting the fact that the body's pH is strictly regulated and that variations from the standard range can be fatal.

Excessive restriction of some food groups or other dietary approaches to change pH may be more detrimental than beneficial. People must prioritize a diverse and well-balanced diet that includes a range of foods high in nutrients to promote general health and well-being.

CHAPTER SIX

Tributes And Success Stories

Adopting the Alkaline Diet has produced excellent results for many people. Testimonials and success stories emphasize the alleged advantages, which include better digestion, more energy, and better skin health.

Although personal tales cannot replace scientific research, they do provide valuable insights into the varied experiences of those who have adopted the Alkaline Diet.

Actual Experiences

Experiences with the Alkaline Diet in real life offer a complex viewpoint on its effects. While some people find it difficult to follow the dietary limitations, others enthusiastically adopt the lifestyle. Examining the difficulties and successes of those who have adopted an Alkaline Diet illuminates the usefulness and viability of sticking to this eating schedule.

Before And Following Transformations

It can be powerful to see people's changes both before and after they follow an alkaline diet.

These metamorphoses frequently display adjustments to body weight, skin tone, and general health.

Analyzing these observable results might provide a visual story about how the Alkaline Diet may affect people's appearance and overall health.

Criticisms And Debates

The Alkaline Diet is not without its detractors and issues, despite its supporters.

Critics contend that substantial pH changes brought about only by diet are ineffective because of the body's built-in regulating systems.

Furthermore, nutrient deficits could result from the diet's restriction. A thorough grasp of the Alkaline Diet and its role in the larger context of nutrition can be obtained by examining both sides of the argument.

In the field of nutrition, people are still interested in and talking about the Alkaline Diet.

People can make more educated decisions about whether to adopt this nutritional strategy into their lifestyles by being aware of its ideas, taking into account real-life experiences, and accepting criticisms.

Even while testimonies and success stories give an idea of the possible advantages, it's important to approach the Alkaline Diet critically and seek the counsel of medical professionals for specific recommendations.

Determining the pH levels in the body is essential to resolving imbalances. Seven is regarded as neutral on the pH scale, which goes from 0 to 14. If the value is less than 7, it is acidic; if it is greater than 7, it is alkaline.

It's commonly said that keeping pH between 7.35 and 7.45, which is slightly alkaline, is optimum.

Symptoms of imbalances include exhaustion, gastrointestinal troubles, skin disorders, and recurrent infections.

For a precise diagnosis, it's crucial to speak with a healthcare provider as these symptoms are not limited to pH imbalances.

It's critical to identify pH imbalance warning indicators to take preventative measures against any health problems. Osteoporosis, acid reflux, and muscular atrophy are among diseases that can result from persistent acidity.

Conversely, long-term alkalinity may cause disorientation, hand tremors, and twitching of the muscles.

Urine pH testing can also reveal information about the acid-base balance in your body.

People who regularly keep an eye out for these warning indicators are better equipped to make educated food judgments.

Consuming foods that support an alkaline environment in the body is the main goal of the alkaline diet. One important element is to emphasize fresh fruits and vegetables, especially those that have a low tendency to create acids. Nuts, seeds, leafy greens, and some grains are frequently advised. On the other hand, it's advisable to limit your consumption of foods that are known to create acid, like dairy, processed meats, and refined sweets. To maintain pH equilibrium, it's also advised to drink plenty of alkaline water. But, it's imperative to keep a balanced approach because drastic dietary adjustments could have unforeseen effects.

Although the Alkaline Diet provides a foundation for encouraging pH balance, consulting a professional is essential. A certified dietician or healthcare professional may evaluate each person's unique health needs and make tailored recommendations.

They can conduct diagnostic tests to find out particular pH values and uncover underlying medical conditions.

Expert advice guarantees that dietary modifications do not jeopardize adequate nutrition and are in line with general health objectives.

Working together with a medical expert guarantees a thorough approach to pH balance, taking into account any underlying health issues.

In conclusion, the Alkaline Diet can be a useful tool for preserving the body's pH equilibrium, but it must be used carefully and intelligently.

To promote overall health and well-being, it's important to recognize the symptoms of pH imbalances, make modest dietary adjustments, and see a specialist.

CHAPTER SEVEN

Sustainability And Extended-Term Dedication:

The Alkaline Diet's sustainability and dedication to adopting it as a long-term lifestyle choice are essential to achieving all of its advantages.

Achieving long-lasting impacts requires ingesting alkaline-forming foods consistently over a protracted period, even though short-term adherence may have some favorable results.

This durable method guarantees that the body adapts gradually, enhancing general health.

The Alkaline Diet must be smoothly incorporated into daily activities to become a lifestyle.

This extends beyond simple dietary limitations and includes deliberate decisions that are in line with the alkaline principles.

A sustainable lifestyle is promoted by including a range of fruits, vegetables, and legumes that are high in alkalis in meals.

Alkaline water further improves the alkaline balance, which is another benefit of maintaining proper hydration and supporting a holistic approach to wellness.

While it can be difficult, maintaining the Alkaline Diet when dining out is not impossible.

Making smart decisions in different eating situations, such as choosing salads with alkaline-rich vegetables, grilling lean proteins, and staying away from highly processed or acidic meals, might help you stick to the diet.

Understanding menu options and communicating dietary preferences to restaurant staff effectively are essential for navigating social situations without jeopardizing the alkaline balance.

Rejoicing In Milestones:

It is essential for motivation and sustained dedication to the Alkaline Diet to recognize and celebrate accomplishments made possible by the diet. Acknowledging these successes—such as achieving a weight reduction objective, feeling more energized, or observing better digestion—confirms the beneficial effects of dietary decisions.

To create a sense of satisfaction and accomplishment on the path toward pH balance, celebrations can take many different forms, such as treating oneself to a special alkaline-friendly meal or sharing successes with a support system.

To sum up, the Alkaline Diet is more than just a food plan; it's a way of living that encompasses a whole lifestyle.

The success of this diet in fostering pH balance and general well-being is attributed to its sustainability, long-term commitment, thoughtful dining selections, and celebration of achievements.

Adopting the Alkaline Diet as a way of life guarantees that the diet's tenets become deeply embedded in routine activities, promoting a more alkaline and healthy internal environment.

On the other hand, the Alkaline Diet suggests consuming fewer foods that cause acidity. Animal products, refined sugars, processed foods, and specific cereals are usually among them. The reasoning behind this is that eating too many acidic foods can cause the body's pH to become too acidic, which supporters claim may be a factor in several health problems.

The Body's Buffer Systems in Balance

Alkaline diet detractors assert that the body has strong buffer systems that closely control pH levels. These systems, which aim to keep the blood's pH within a certain range, include the respiratory and renal systems. Although food can affect urine pH, its effect on the body's total pH may be limited.

There is conflicting evidence about the direct impact of food pH on blood pH.

Alleged Advantages of an Alkaline Diet

Alkaline diet proponents assert several health advantages, such as increased immunity, weight loss, and increased energy.

Many contend that an alkaline environment within the body is less favorable for the emergence of specific illnesses, such as cancer and osteoporosis. However, the scientific data backing up these assertions is frequently scant and ambiguous.

The Alkaline Diet has come under fire for lacking strong scientific backing for its assertions. Strict adherence to this diet may also result in nutritional imbalances because it restricts several vital nutrients and acid-forming foods. People thinking about adopting this diet must speak with medical specialists to make sure they get the nourishment they need.

Conclusion

the Alkaline Diet emphasizes the harmony of acidic and alkaline foods, offering a comprehensive strategy for overall health. The diet's specific health claims are not well supported by scientific research, even though its principles support the goal of maintaining a slightly alkaline pH in the body. People must proceed cautiously while making dietary adjustments, taking into account their unique health requirements and consulting medical professionals for advice.

the Main Ideas

The Alkaline Diet places a strong emphasis on eating foods that generate an alkaline environment to keep the body's pH level in balance.

The body's ideal pH level is slightly alkaline, and maintaining pH balance is essential for general health.

Foods that form an alkaline medium include fruits, vegetables, nuts, seeds, and some grains; foods that form an acid medium, such as processed foods and animal products, should be consumed in moderation.

There is conflicting evidence about the direct effects of diet on blood pH because the body has strong buffer systems that control pH levels.

Advocates assert a variety of health advantages, but there is frequently scant scientific proof to back up these assertions.

The diet has come under fire for possible nutritional imbalances and a lack of solid scientific support.

Continue on Your Path to pH Balance

It is crucial to approach food decisions with knowledge as you make your way towards pH equilibrium. Take into account speaking with medical experts, and keep in mind each person's unique dietary requirements.

Recall that attaining and preserving pH balance is a complex process including a holistic approach to general health and wellbeing.

www.ingramcontent.com/pod-product-compliance
Lightning Source LLC
Chambersburg PA
CBHW060804260726
48660CB00002B/771